Table Of Contents

Introduction

Yoga is something else for most people. They are different and practitioners have different expectations when they start. That is very good. Whether your goal is more relief, a firmer and more muscular body, or pain relief, yoga is for you. This book will serve as a guide.

The philosophy of yoga has existed for 5,000 years. This is an undeniable lasting force. Yoga is not just an "exercise", it is a philosophy, a way of thinking like a religion. In ancient India, the word yoga meant unity. It refers to the unity of the whole self - mind, body, and spirit. This oneness can be achieved through physical positions, often called asanas, even though the asana is just one of many yoga lessons. These positions are designed to increase mind and body awareness, making yoga a natural consequence of meditation.

Researchers have now discovered the many benefits of yoga. While it can increase spirituality, it also has the potential to heal many diseases and ailments, especially stress, immune system diseases, and heart problems. It also provides more flexibility that can reverse the aging process.

The strongest yoga exercises are considered cardiovascular exercises. With the right diet, you can lose weight. Gentle types of yoga do not have cardiovascular benefits, so be sure to do more exercise.

Why did people become interested in yoga? The most common reason is to improve flexibility and fitness. In addition to the physical benefits, yoga also increases the strength of the mind and creates a path for spiritual enlightenment.

For many, it is the spiritual awakening that makes yoga an essential part of their lives. It's a slow but amazing development and an opportunity for personal growth. The essence of yoga is always to be a better version of oneself.

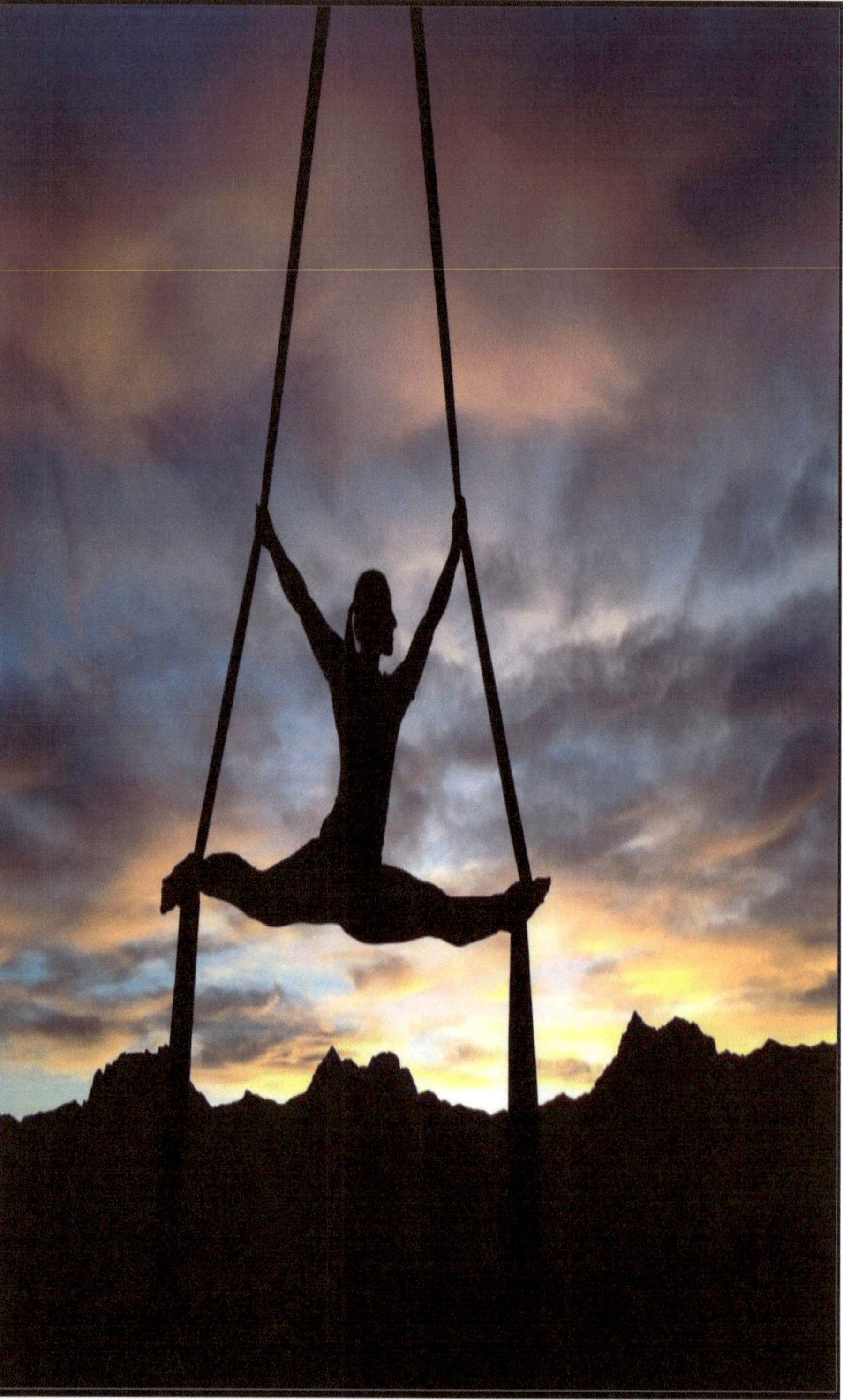

Chapter 01 – What is the Science of Yoga?

People have been practicing yoga for thousands of years. While the original goal was to rise to a more spiritual level, yoga has been shown to benefit people in general. Modern scientific research has shown many general health benefits of the yoga lifestyle.

Yes, yoga improves the body, but shocking scientific research shows that it also changes the brain. It is a better version of oneself and making contact with the real, real self because the brain is silent. It keeps us focused today. When mathematical yoga began, it spread throughout the day as greater compassion and knowledge became part of our lives.

Yoga does not provide countless riches, although the physical benefits are remarkable. The world is full of abundance, which we mostly ignore. The real beauty of yoga is that it strengthens us to this day, connects us to the abundance that is in our understanding. We have a better and more satisfying life at hand when we walk and just accept what is available.

Every yoga position, which often involves stretching, has a purpose and an advantage. Practitioners are aware of stress and learn to release it. Yoga positions are very specific and perfection comes with practice, but that is not the ultimate goal. Yoga involves a lot of stretching, but above all, it creates balance by increasing flexibility and strength. Whatever yoga you practice, heal your body and mind.

Yoga is extremely diverse and individual, which makes it important to work at your own level of comfort. Don't use the person next to you in class as a guide, or even the teacher. Work the poses in the best way for you. This isn't a speed contest, and you have nothing to prove. Yoga is a lifetime commitment, not a competition.

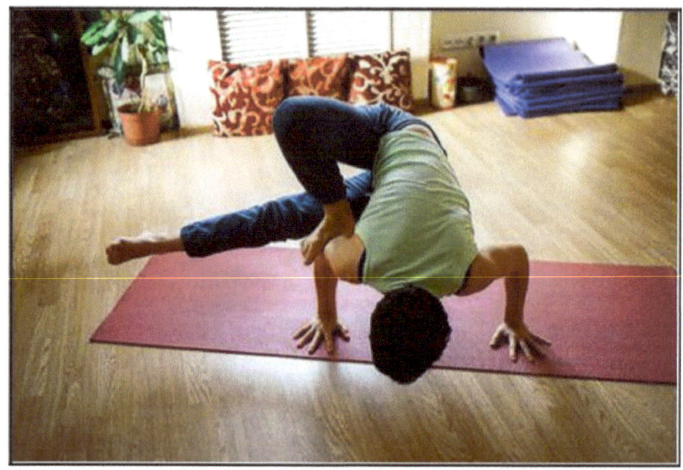

Even if you are not used to practicing, you can practice yoga. You may not be as flexible as the others, but you will get there. Yoga has always been continuous work and not a competition. Even if it is a physical practice, yoga will inevitably affect your mental side. It unites the mind and body to become one. Research conducted in the 20th century found many physical benefits to practicing yoga.

Relief from Stress

Our lives are filled with daily stressors, and we know that stress can cause tremendous damage to the body and mind. The boss wants to talk, your spouse is upset, the mortgage is overdue, and the kids want the keys to the car. Just another typical day. Holding yoga poses, stretching muscles, being focused on the presents, and breathing deeply and slowly helps us achieve a state of greater relaxation and harmony. We are able to consciously choose our response to stress instead of being at its mercy. Remaining calm under difficult circumstances is a choice, and yoga can provide the tools.

Yoga and Pain Relief

Studies have proven that practicing yoga can provide tremendous relief for people suffering from multiple sclerosis, arthritis, and other chronic conditions. We'll discuss its amazing effect on the auto-immune system and cardio system at greater length in other chapters.

Yoga and Breathing

Yoga combines physical movements with breathing. Slower, deeper breathing can alleviate stress.

Yoga and Flexibility

Yoga involves a lot a stretching, which strengthens muscles. Since yoga impacts the entire body, flexibility and elasticity from head to toe. It also loosens tight, tense muscles and helps us become more relaxed.

Yoga and Weight Control

Yoga does not burn as many calories as other exercises. However, it increases awareness of the body. People who practice yoga are more aware of what they eat and how such foods affect their health. This often leads to better, healthier eating habits and natural weight loss.

Yoga and blood circulation

If your blood cannot supply your body and brain with the right oxygen, your health will suffer. You need good circulation for brain function, energy, and cell growth. Slow circulation can cause nerve and tissue damage, blood clots, dizziness, and other problems. Complete stretching in most yoga positions can improve blood circulation. The camel position described in this book is a great way to improve blood circulation.

Yoga and Cardio health

For patients who have undergone heart surgery, depression and anxiety can be a natural outcomes. Yoga can help manage this type of postoperative stress. It can also lower blood pressure, which serves as a preventative measure for heart health. The specific benefits of the heart are discussed in a separate chapter. No rush - take your time Achieving these benefits will take some time.

Yoga is not a two-week miracle program. So when you start yoga, allow enough time for the results to show. You should see a big difference in about two months. Whatever your reason for practicing yoga, you need to consider improvement in all aspects of your being.

Chapter 02 – The Ancient History of Yoga

Yoga has become a trend nowadays as practitioners wear their yoga pants and mats to popular yoga studios to attend their weekly yoga classes. What most of these yoga trends do not know is the long history of yoga dating back to antiquity in India and its spiritual roots.

Most of what we think about yoga did not begin until 150 years ago. While people today practice yoga for their health, their roots are associated with rich spiritualism that lasts a lifetime to embrace.

For ancient yogis, yoga was a way of life. The mention of yoga first appears around 1500 BC. in Hindu literature. In early writings, in traditional Sanskrit, the term yoga, meaning joke, always referred to a mortal warrior who ascended to heaven and attained a higher power.

The original concept of yoga clearly elevates its advantages to a higher level in order to connect individuals with the universe as a whole. Yoga was not a specific discipline for ancient Buddhists.

It grows out of a desire to achieve spiritual goals and to control the mind and body to achieve them.

These spiritual leaders acknowledge that one is wrong, but they are always able to make progress by changing bad thinking.

They recognize the power of the mind to bring inner peace and alleviate suffering by expanding individual consciousness and openness to new ideas. He already understands the basics of mind/body connection.

Yoga, including meditation, has become and still is a search for knowledge. Ancient practitioners rightly believed that knowledge would lead to a higher level of knowledge and existence.

The ancient scriptures describe a specific level of being with the addition of knowledge that will take the practitioner to the next, higher level. It is considered a process that involves learning for most lifelong learning. Yoga, the physical part of receiving enlightenment, is to pave the way for spiritual meditation in nature.

The physical aspect of yoga began to appear in 500 AD. In the third century, yoga was a recognized Buddhist practice that involved spiritual search through meditation. This was the classical period in which Vyasa's writings introduced all the basic yoga sutras and introduced yoga as a condition for a longer life.

Practicing yoga has been a recognized practice for many centuries to achieve essential personal qualities, even though it is far from current. It is to help "overcome" and exaggerate human suffering more thoughtfully. It is also used to expand or deepen consciousness as a path to personal enlightenment. Yoga is seen as a way to overcome destiny and regain self-control.

The beginning of training and mind control was clear. Until the 15th century, when the West was in a state of constant struggle and war, Eastern Buddhism focused on peace of mind. The difference between the Western and Eastern mentalities is becoming clearer. During this time, the emphasis on yoga shifts from overcoming pain to achieving a higher state of life. Man himself has become a god.

In the eighth century, hatha yoga, a combination of pose and meditation, became a practice. This was the beginning of the "modern" yoga we know today. Yoga, an ancient spiritual endeavor of Buddhism, did not reach the West until the end of the 19th century. This is in line with the interest in Indian culture as a whole through the thriving herb trade.

Western culture was interested in the writings of Swami Vivekananda, a monk who traveled to Europe and introduced intelligence to Buddhist spiritual writings, especially the 4th-century yoga sutras, which involved clearing the mind of unwanted thoughts and learning to focus on one thing. Yoga, as we know it today, became popular in the United States in the 1940s, when young Americans began taking yoga classes. In the 1980s, the well-known health benefits of yoga increased its popularity, although most practitioners considered exercise to be more physical than mental.

In the 21st century, the number of American yoga practitioners increased from 4 million at the turn of the century to 20 million in 2011. This increase in popularity is mainly due to additional scientific studies of the many benefits of yoga, especially stress relief. Mentally or not, people want to improve their health.

However, many people still strive for mental and physical heights. Yoga offers both. While mastering the physical aspects of yoga is important, it is equally important not to forget the spiritual benefits. Yoga is more than just posting beautiful selfies on Instagram.

Thousands of years ago, yoga was preparation for spiritual enlightenment through meditation. He has to prepare the body and relax it for meditation practice. It is important not to forget that. To reach your spiritual side, remember the seven spiritual laws of yoga:

1.   You have unlimited potential. The goal of yoga is to achieve a high level of awareness.

2.   The universe is full of abundance. Accept, learn to give.

3.   Understand the universal law of cause and effect, known as karma. Your actions, both positive and negative, will be eliminated to the same extent.

4.   Don't resist the forces of life. Your desires will manifest themselves if you can't resist..

5.   Explain what your wishes and purpose are.

6.   Stop fighting and stay open to all opportunities that come your way.

7.   Find out what your real meaning in life is.

The meditation discussed in the last chapter of this book can help you achieve the spiritual laws of yoga.

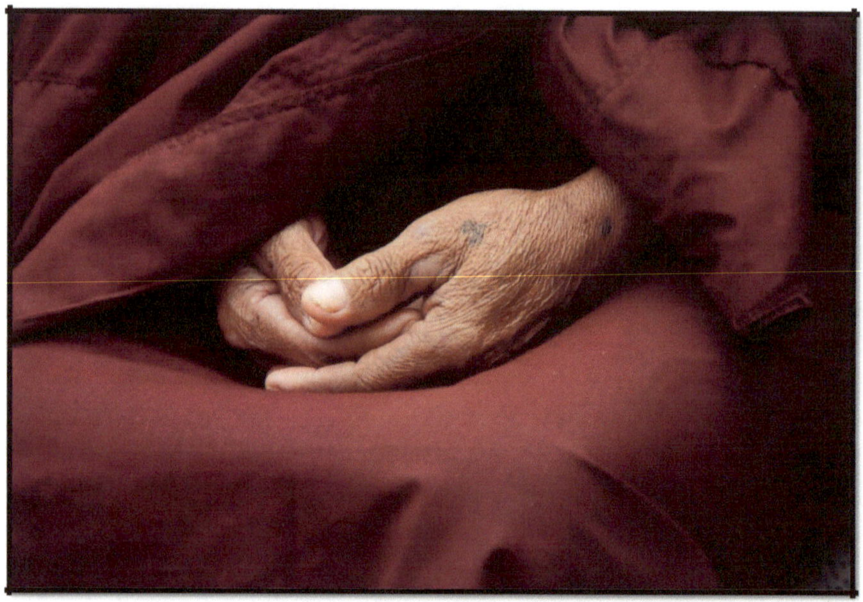

Chapter 03 - Establishing the Mind/Body Connection with Yoga

The purpose of yoga has always been to connect the mind with the body. That's what Buddhists thought thousands of years ago. Even in the past, it is clear that as the mind, and body work together, they themselves become healthier, more thoughtful, and able to function at a higher level.

But how are the mind and body connected? People who are aware of their thoughts and feelings can better deal with the stresses and difficulties of life. They create better and healthier relationships. In the end, he believes in his ability to succeed.

We all face setbacks. It's how we handle them that makes the difference. Emotional wellbeing is rarely a constant, however. Unexpected events can lead to depression, anxiety, stress, and confusion.

Unemployment, physical injury, death, the injury of someone we love, or the end of a relationship can cause emotional turmoil. Even positive events, such as a new home, wedding, or new job, can cause fear when confronted with an unknown person.

When our mind experiences problems, the body responds immediately. As if you needed a reminder, the body is here to tell you that everything is wrong. The body does this in many ways such as developing high blood pressure, ulceration, insomnia, and so on. All of these symptoms are physical manifestations of a worried mind. Whether we realize it or not, the mind and body function as a team.

So, where does yoga come into play?

As yoga increases our knowledge of the mind, we become more aware of basic emotions and thoughts. This allows us to express and recognize them instead of leaving them buried and upset. The correct expression of negative emotions allows us to deal with them and throw them behind our heads.

If we deal effectively with the negative ones, we will recognize the more positive aspects of our lives. Sometimes we are so overwhelmed that we don't see anything better or positive, even if it's around us. Yoga provides the necessary balance. Yes, work can be stressful, but we find that there is more to our lives. It's a healthy view that improves our overall quality of life when we need it.

A healthy connection between mind and body gives us the ability to deal with adversity as we become stronger. Strength is a skill that can be learned and developed. It prevents us from falling victim to circumstances and gives us more control over our lives. We can strengthen the condition by relaxing and developing a calmer look.

Yoga and meditation are valuable tools to control our thoughts, emotions, and lives in general. When we have everything under control, we sleep better, eat healthier, and communicate with others at a higher level.

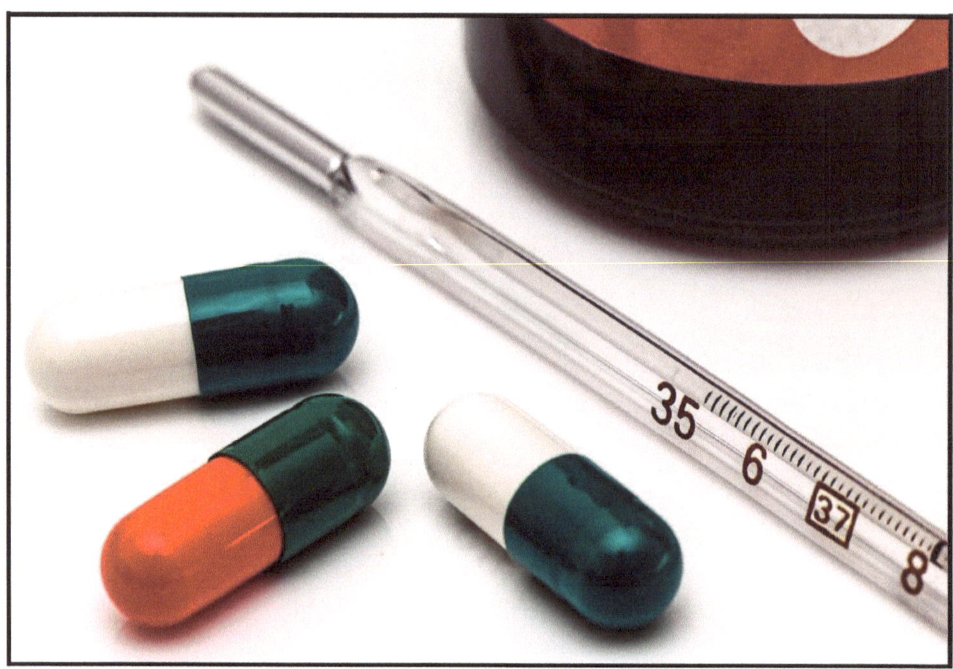

Our emotional health often affects our immune system, as we will see in another chapter. A weakened immune system can make the body prone to colds, inflammation, and infections.

Many of the ways in which the mind affects the body became clearer in the 20th century when repeated research revealed how stress and emotions can inevitably intersect and connect. Fortunately, modern physicians are more integrated with their patients' health. Many others recommend yoga and meditation not only for stress but for cardiovascular disease, everything is fine.

Discuss the general benefits of yoga with your doctor. Regardless of your mental and physical health, it can always be improved.

Chapter 04 – Yoga – Strength and Flexibility

Strength training, usually in the form of weightlifting such as Cross Fit, has become popular. Women especially appreciate a more outlined, muscular, and stronger body.

Increasing physical strength is important to prevent osteoporosis and natural muscle loss during aging. Strong muscles help keep joints healthy and prevent injuries.

While the benefits of strength training are obvious, some people doubt whether yoga exercises allow for increased strength and muscle. This can be especially true for male athletes, who perceive yoga as a "female" activity. But can yoga really strengthen muscles?

It depends on the type of yoga you practice. Some yoga lessons are supposed to be gentle. Restorative yoga falls into this category. This only makes them less effective; It just means that many people, especially the elderly, will enjoy the benefits of yoga. As we have already mentioned, yoga is for everyone.

However, there are yoga exercises that are hard and demanding and can be difficult for a strong man. Poses like Planks and Warrior require full-body support and can definitely improve muscle and strength. These positions can strengthen the whole body, not just the specific muscles that are supposed to train when weightlifting. For maximum results, there may be positions with small dumbbells. Therefore, yoga can be better at building strength than other types of exercise.

Ashtanga and Vinyasas yoga can increase strength through multiple repetition positions, especially on the upper body and legs. In addition, holding positions for longer periods of time, such as up to two minutes per pose, is good muscle regeneration. Keep in mind that it takes a while to create such a state.

But building muscle is an individual goal. How many muscles are enough? For most muscle workers, weights can definitely help you get faster results. Many people use yoga and weightlifting to dramatically increase volume.

Unlike strengthening, yoga is not focused on the body. It's more than just an exercise.

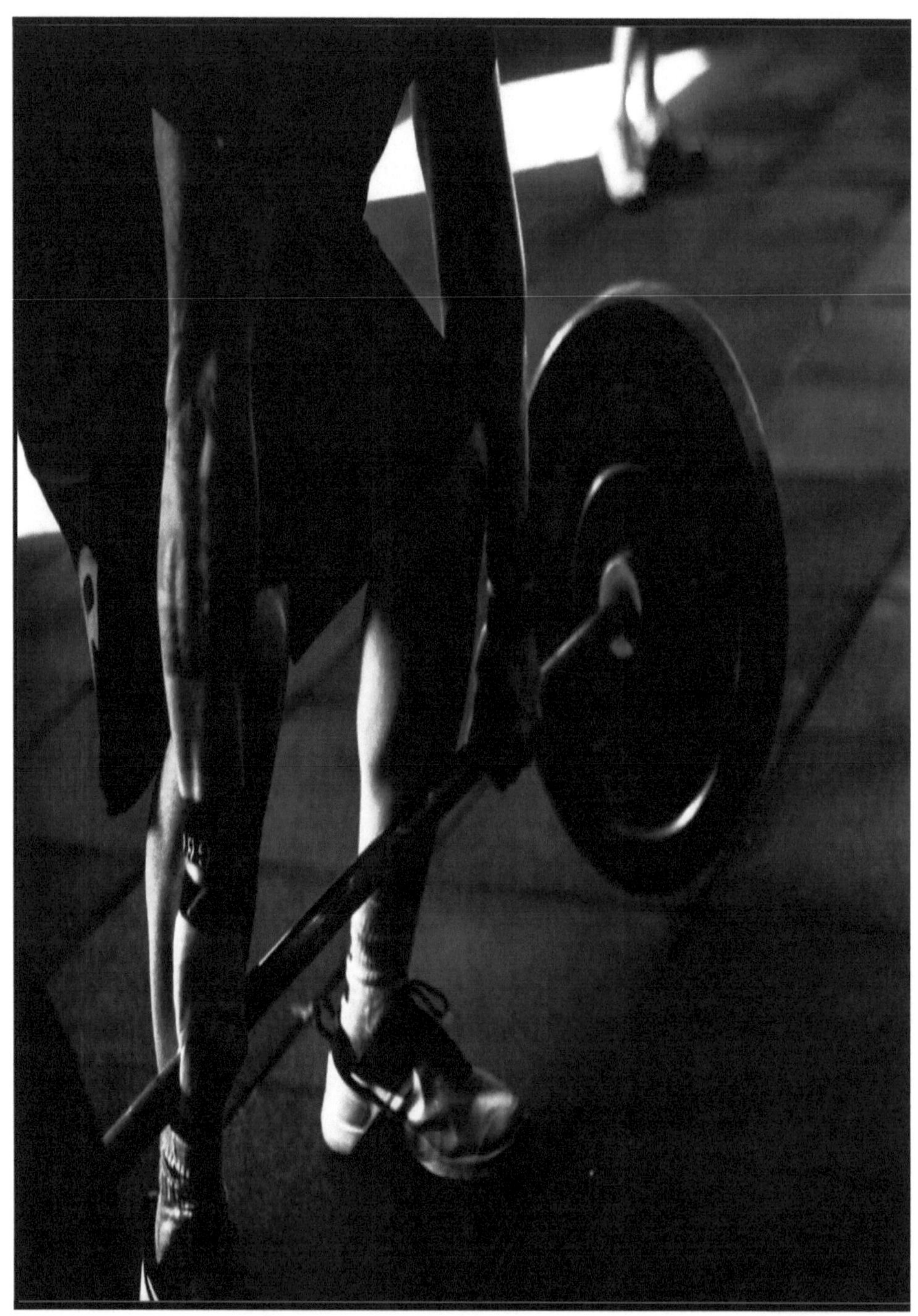

With weightlifting, you can build muscle forever by simply adding more weights. If you want, you can build separate muscles, such as your torso-sized legs. With yoga, you build strength in a more balanced way, because all muscles, big and small, are built. Weight is energy instead of volume. Your body becomes stronger and allows you to use this energy in all physical activities such as lifting, twisting, and bending. Instead of being a more muscular person, you will become a stronger individual.

You can include other exercises in your yoga program. But yoga alone, if you practice it regularly, will continue to improve your body and increase strength and flexibility.

Yoga sections are widely known for improving flexibility. Flexibility and balance are especially important as we age and become more prone to injury. Many people think that you have to be flexible before you start practicing yoga, but the opposite is true. You can start yoga in any physical state and continue to improve your flexibility.

There are three specific parts of the body that are always tense: the thighs, shoulders, and buttocks. We spend a lot of time inactive and sitting, and these muscles can become irreversible when not exercising.

Stretching Aila Yoga can greatly increase your flexibility if you train these muscle groups properly. As always, do not stretch the muscles until the pain. Stretch to the limit of your comfort and you will soon see the result

Now let's talk about another muscle that can be immutable, the brain. Yes, the brain is really a muscle. When you have strict attitudes, such as things that only need to be done one way, you limit your mental strength. Maybe your mind is constantly coming up with certain problems and you don't see a reason to investigate them further. The purpose of yoga is to release your mental strength. It's about changing all aspects of your life. Yoga is a big four-letter word.

The combination of yoga and meditation opens the mind to new ideas and ways to do things. It inspires curiosity. Many people stick to the fear of old, traditional ideas. Yoga has rid of this fear and opens up new, life-improving possibilities.

When it comes to yoga, you will soon enjoy a more flexible body, such as a mind that will be open, flexible, and interesting.

Chapter 05 - Managing Weight with Yoga

It is a well-known fact that exercise, especially aerobic lessons, has a positive effect on heart health. Heart disease is a major killer because plaque in the arteries begins to block natural blood flow. More than 600,000 people in the United States have died of heart disease, but it is completely preventable. The main causes are smoking, obesity, poor diet, and inactivity. The yoga lifestyle usually eliminates all four of these factors to ensure better cardio health.

Many people avoid the word "exercise", they think they have gone crazy or run on the track in aerobics classes. These exercises are absolutely beneficial, but they are not the only ones that help us maintain a healthy heart and a long life.

Yoga, along with gentle but challenging positions, can provide the benefits of aerobic exercise in an easier way.

There are many studies that compare yoga without exercise and compare yoga with regular aerobic exercise.

Compared to people who did not exercise or exercise, those who practiced yoga showed a clear and substantial improvement in heart health. They lost weight and achieved a significant reduction in blood pressure. Their cholesterol levels have also improved.

These results are expected. The surprise comes when people who practice yoga are compared to people who do regular aerobics. There were no significant differences between the two weight loss groups, cholesterol level, or blood pressure. The yoga group achieved the same level of benefits as the aerobics group.

A group of independent researchers, the Cochrane Collaboration, confirmed the results but showed that the amount of time spent each week practicing yoga can have a long-term effect. People who attend a weekly yoga class have fewer benefits than those who practice yoga several times a week or every day.

Many Americans suffer from atrial fibrillation, an irregular heartbeat that can cause high blood pressure, stress and obesity. As with conventional heart disease, atrial fibrillation can be prevented.

The University of Kansas study used a group of 52 patients with atrial fibrillation and included them in two weekly yoga classes for several months. The results of the study found that participants enjoyed improved heart rate and reduced anxiety and blood pressure.

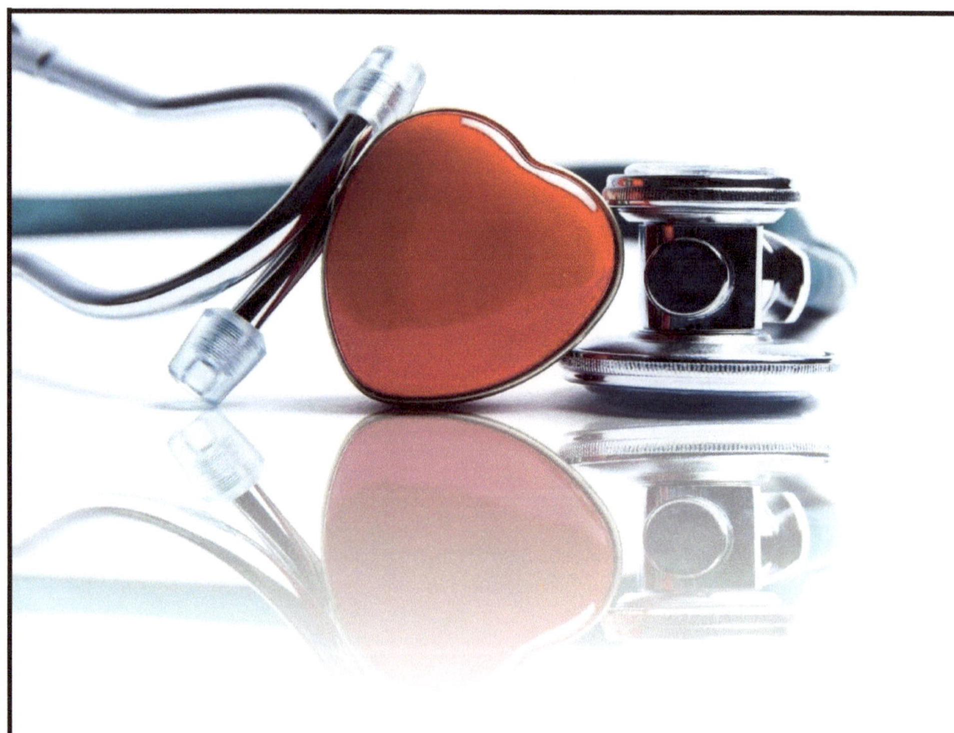

Recent evidence suggests that yoga if practiced regularly, can provide the same cardio benefits as traditional aerobic exercise.

Transcendental meditation is a type of yoga meditation that we will discuss in a later chapter. A study by the American Heart Association found that transcendental meditation can reduce the risk of cardiovascular death in almost half of the patients with heart problems.

Another study by the Medical College of Wisconsin included half of the group of patients with high blood pressure in the group of transcendental meditations and the other half taking blood pressure medications. The meditation group practiced 20 minutes a day for up to five years.

The study showed that almost half of the meditation group had a reduction in heart problems compared to the medication group.

Additional studies have been performed. However, there is clear evidence that yoga has a significant positive effect on heart health.

Yoga and Weight Management

While there are easier ways to lose weight, yoga can help you lose a few pounds.

Yoga does not burn the same amount of calories as aerobic exercise. An hour of yoga will burn about 150 calories, and an hour's walk will burn more than 300 calories. But losing weight is more than burning calories, although yoga provides a healthy workout. However, there is another, more subtle, influence.

Yoga raises awareness of our body and the food we use to burn it. If your diet consists of burgers and fries, an improved mind-body connection will increase the toxicity of certain foods and allow you to achieve healthier and life-saving options. Toxic foods may be less attractive. This means that most people come for a salad instead of a burger.

If you want to lose weight using your yoga regimen, choose more powerful yoga lessons such as Kundalini Yoga and Yin Yoga.

Chapter 06 – Different Types of Yoga

There are so many different types of yoga disciplines that choosing one can be confusing. Let diversity not stop you from plunging into the yoga pool. There are several types of yoga aimed at beginners and this is your best way to learn about the moves.

Also, keep in mind that the teacher can create or disrupt the experience. If a particular lesson does not suit you, it may be a teacher instead of yoga. Research until you find your perfect fit for yoga.

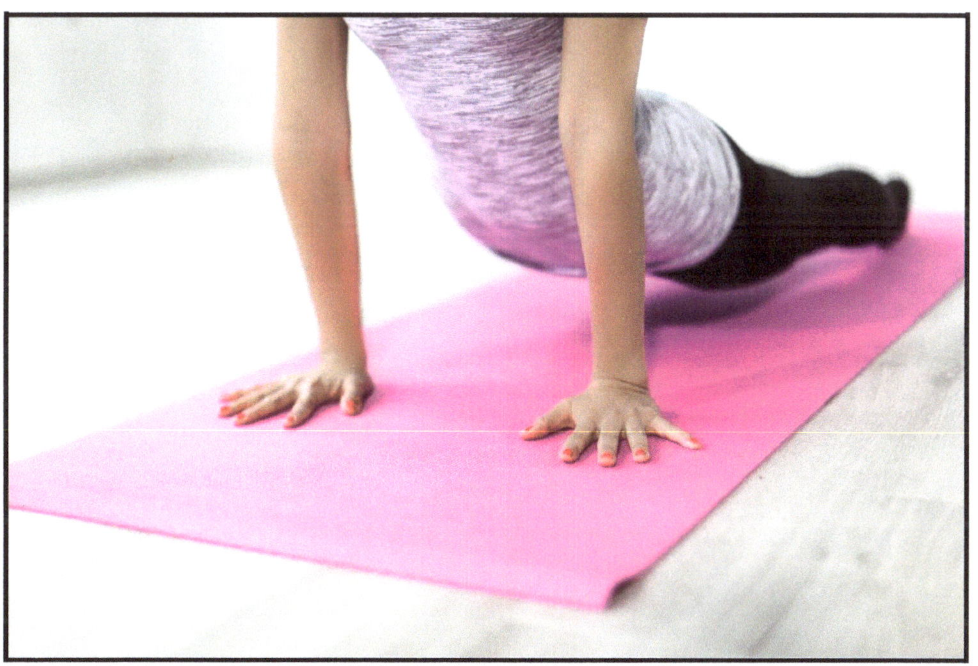

To start yoga at home, you will need a mat, a yoga pad or towel if needed, and a strap that you can use as a plug in some bent positions.

Hatha Yoga

Hatha yoga is the most common form of yoga and probably the most difficult to explain. Depending on the teacher, the lessons may be slow and easy, but some may be more difficult. To make sure that a particular Hatha lesson is right for you, visit the lessons as a guest before you register.

Hatha yoga consists of gentle movements without continuous flow between positions. This makes it easier for beginners to learn the basics. It is highly adaptable to individual needs and physical conditions and is a great way to increase strength and flexibility while reducing the risk of injury.

This is the best place to start and learn basic positions before moving on to more difficult movements and positions. The emphasis is on maintaining position and maintaining balance. Hatha yoga is a slow movement, so if your goal is to move fast and sweaty, this is not the best option. The benefits of hatha yoga are to reduce stress and blood pressure as the body learns to relax.

Vinyasa Yoga

Vinyasa yoga has a faster pace than Hatha, and positions can move faster with each other, instead of dancing steps. Every movement is related to inhaling and exhaling, so the breathing movement is interconnected. The mind remains focused and present. There is no strict order of poses and teachers can "mix and compare" and change routine. So if a particular type of vinyasa doesn't appeal to you, you want something different. Vinyasa yoga is less gentle than Hatha and lowers the limits of flexibility and strength.

It provides good cardio exercise because your body is constantly on the move, except when the dog is resting. You will definitely sweat.

Iyengar Yoga
Iyengar Yoga is an extension of Hatha Yoga that specifically focuses on body tuning
and can be very beneficial. This increases flexibility due to slow stretching
movements over a period of time. These moments have meditative properties.
Maintains muscles and calms the mind. Better balance can strengthen muscles,
help with pain and improve posture. Iyengar yoga covers the whole body and
improves blood circulation and digestion. With a better and healthier body often
comes a better lifestyle choice.
This type of yoga can use chairs, straps, or other props to improve posture. It is
perfectly suitable for beginners.

Ashtanga Yoga
Ashtanga yoga is more structured than other asanas. There are a number of moves, a
total of six, and each series must be mastered before proceeding to the next.
Ashtanga yoga is not for beginners. It is a challenge for strength, endurance, and
flexibility; therefore, it is best to begin ashtanga yoga after some acquaintance
with other yoga disciplines.Ashtanga affects the whole body, so the results come quickly.
It takes effort, and most Ashtanga practitioners do the exercises every day. It can take
years to master each series. Patients will love Ashtanga because it requires repeating the
same positions. There is no difference until you reach the next level.

Bikram Yoga
There are 26 positions that need to be completed in a structured order for each Bikram
session that lasts 1 hour and a half. Bikram's turn is that he trains at a temperature of
105 degrees. You sweat and need to stay hydrated. Heat, of course, adds another
challenge. It also adds benefits such as removing toxins from the body.

Hot Yoga
As the name suggests, Hot Yoga is also performed in a room full of high temperatures.
This differs from Bikram because Hot Yoga has no structure without 26 specific
positions. This is suitable for beginners, but consider another challenge posed by heat.

Kundalini Yoga

Kundalini uses meditation to stimulate the body. Its effects on the mind are extremely

strong because it increases knowledge and strengthens your inner self so that you can be

more real. It reminds me of the beginning of yoga in its search for spiritual heights.

Kundalini yoga mixes breathing and songs.

Yin Yoga

Yin Yoga combines physical and mental and is specially designed to stimulate and soothe a busy mind.

The advantage of regular exercise is a feeling of calm, reduced stress, improved blood circulation and flexibility, and greater joint mobility. The principle of Yin Yoga is the concept of yin and yang in Taoism, which seeks to balance all differences in nature.

The exercises are performed on the floor and include holding poses for a long time. It can affect the lower body, especially the thighs, legs, and spine. Poses can be done in five minutes or more.

In a world that is constantly being stimulated, the mind is easily overcome and overcome. It is considered "normal" to the extent that people are proud of a type-A personality. They are full of a sense of urgency to always move.

The body cannot relax and the mind cannot be silent. Yin yoga brings a balance of mind and body. The long pose stretches the tissues and strengthens the body while allowing for mental awareness. A large amount of energy is used to suppress unwanted thoughts and emotions. Yin yoga releases this energy.

Restorative Yoga

Restorative yoga will restore your mind and body. It is easy, slow moving, with positions held for a long time to achieve a state of complete relaxation. You can use props such as blocks to help you maintain your position.

Chapter 07 - Attaining Better Immunity with Yoga Poses

A healthy immune system is the body's first defense against inflammation and disease, from cancer to the flu. For your immune system to work properly, it must be balanced. This means that cells, organs and tissues work together to act as an army, ready to defend the body against intruders such as bacteria and other contaminants. The immune system produces antibodies that help cure infections and remove toxins from the body.

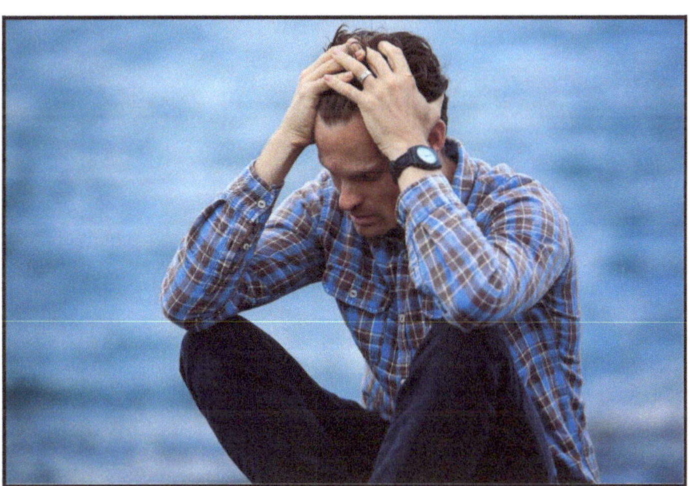

Have you ever wondered why some people catch every mistake that causes beats while others seem immune? A period of stress can make our immune system even more vulnerable. So the healthier our immune system is, the easier it will be to overcome the effects of bacteria, germs and toxins. Healthy cells immediately reach our defenses and attack the attackers. These useful soldiers are white blood cells.

Yoga is a natural relaxant and stress reliever and is a great way to keep our immune system at an optimal level. It provides much-needed relief in times of stress.

Researchers have studied the link between yoga and the immune system. A study in the Journal of Behavioral Medicine showed that yoga can help reduce inflammation. In 15 separate tears, the researchers examined whether practicing yoga can affect inflammation. Most studies have been done at speed, according to Hatha. The results of these studies show the formula that yoga reduces inflammation and has a positive effect on the body.

The best yoga programs are those that last up to 12 weeks in lessons per hour. Consistent practice is the key to success.

In addition to inflammation, there are specific asanas that help reduce the irritation of the common cold, such as the position of the turtle.

Tortoise Pose

Sit with your toes pressed against the floor. Spread your legs. Inhale and lower your body close to the floor while breathing. Feel the stretching of the spine and inner legs. Hold the pose for 10 breaths. Put your hands under your knees and hold each leg. Depending on how flexible you are, you can lean forward as much as possible, but don't force it. Inhale to widen your chest, and inhale as you lower your body.

When the cavities become clogged, Downward Dog (see Poses) can help reduce overload. This downward bending position can also help with infections because it depletes the lungs.

Camel Pose for Bronchitis

If you suffer from clogged bronchi, the Camel position may open your body so that you can breathe better.

Camel Pose can also help with neck and back pain. Camel Pose can be hard on your back, so talk to your doctor before you start.

Start by stretching your back with Cobra Pose. This is a very good warm-up and can prevent overweight spine. Camel Pose is a difficult position that you will immediately master, so do not rush and work your way up to the extension of the whole back.

Remember that no yoga position is forced. Kneel on the mat with your hands on your hips. Insert the ankle and push the tail bone to the floor. Lean forward the pan. If necessary, place your hands on the coccyx.

This is a fast-changing camel pose. Once you have done this, you can turn your hands back and hold your heels. Stay in the Camel position for 60 seconds or until you feel uncomfortable.

Whatever yoga you practice, it can help strengthen your immune system. Multiple forward and reverse rotations are especially useful in giving your system the hand it needs.

Yoga Poses

There are approximately 84 asanas, and this chapter will introduce you to a few of the basic ones. A few dos and don't before you start your journey:

- Do wear comfortable clothes.

- Don't practice asanas on a full stomach.

- Don't force any poses to the point of pain. Yoga is painless and should feel comfortable. Your flexibility and strength will improve with practice.

Mountain Pose

This is your starting point for all standing positions. It may seem easy to just stand there, but it's designed to make you feel simple.

Stand straight with your feet naturally apart. Stick all ten fingers to the ground. Raise your knees and inner legs to the upper height. Place the stomach and lift the chest. Lower your shoulders.

Keep your palms close to your body. Inhale and feel your chest even more. Hold the pose for 5 seconds.

Cat Pose

This is one of the most popular yoga positions. Bend your arms and knees and make sure your knees are sitting on your shoulders. Keep your head neutral.

Inhale and lift your spine up and your head down. Inhale and lower your spine and raise your head to the ceiling. Do it several times.

Downward Dog

Another favorite animal pose among yoga enthusiasts, this pose provides a wonderful stretch.

Lower your hands and knees and place your hands on the floor.

Inhale and raise your knees. Your heels will lift. Raise the cob to the ceiling.

While breathing, lower your heels to the floor and straighten your knees until your feet are straight. Keep your arms strong as you straighten them.

Warrior Pose

Exhale and spread your legs about 4 feet apart. Raise your hands until they are directly on the floor.

Move the left foot 60 degrees to the right and the right foot 90 degrees to the right. Heels need to be adjusted.

Inhale and bend the right knee towards the right knee. In practice, your right foot will be parallel to the floor.

Lift your ribs and hold your left foot. You should feel the back of your left leg stretching all the way to your abdomen. Take your palms.

Hold this position for 30 seconds. Inhale, push the back heel to the floor and lift and straighten the right knee.

Take a deep breath turn your legs and repeat the exercise.

Extended Puppy Pose

Breathe and put your hand back to your heel. Keep your arms in front and your elbows above the ground.

With your fist over your heels, lower your forehead to the floor. Feel your spine stretch. Breathe in the spine and hold the pose for 30 seconds.

Inhale and put your hand back to your heels. Keep your arms in front and your elbows above the ground.

With your fist over your heels, lower your forehead to the floor. Feel your spine stretch. Breathe in the spine and hold the pose for 30 seconds.

Triangle

The triangle stretches and restores the whole body. Stand with your feet apart. Raise both arms to shoulder length.

Rotate the right leg 90 degrees and the other leg 45 degrees. Lower your right hand to your knee or, if you can, touch your pelvis. Raise your other hand to the ceiling.

Hold the pose for 8 breaths and then repeat the exercise on the other side

Cobra

Lie down on the floor. Your legs are stretched without touching. Rest your hands on your palms under your shoulders, pointing your fingers forward.

Inhale as you pull your chest and head up as you straighten your arms and continue to grasp the floor. Hold your shoulders as you lift your chest. Do not use unnatural lifting.

Hold the Cobra Pose for up to 30 seconds.

Tree Pose

The Tree Pose helps achieve and maintain balance while standing on one foot. This is a great asana for beginners.

Start by standing with your feet together. Raise your right foot as high as you can, to the upper left thigh. Lift your hands and press the palms together. Keep looking ahead while maintaining your balance.

Plank Pose

Move to the Plank Pose from the Downward Dog. Inhale and lift your torso forward until your elbows are on the floor.

Press your lower arms into the floor and gaze at the floor.

Hold the Plank Pose for 30 seconds and work up to 1 minute. This pose is designed to build strength. Keep breathing and make sure your shoulders are relaxed.

Chapter 08 - How to Get Started

Doing Yoga?

When you begin your yoga journey, you need to keep in mind how important your mental behavior is to success. With exercise comes physical dexterity and flexibility. But to start training, you need the right mentality.

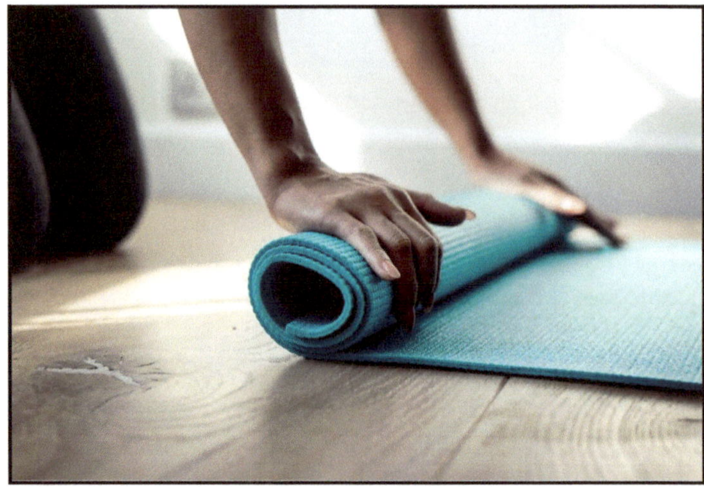

For a beginner, this can be very confusing. Just choosing the right yoga outfit can hurt your head! How do you decide which yoga practice is best for you?

So start with relaxation and consider the following as your plan for successful yoga practice:

Rid Yourself of Expectations

If you are looking at photos of yoga positions and decide that you cannot achieve this kind of agility, keep in mind that it will inevitably take years, perhaps decades, for the model to reach this level. He was specially selected for his skills.

Yoga is not about achieving the perfect pose. It's all about improving breathing and tuning. Step by step and more will follow. If you cannot touch your toes, touch your knees instead. Remove all the expectations you have and start with an open mind. Yoga is not condemning; this is not competition. Regardless of the practice, you will obviously proceed.

Age and body shape are mental limitations and have no effect on your ability to start yoga. If you can't do a certain position, there are dozens of other positions that you can handle.

Find the right teacher

As you know in high school and college, the right teacher can make a huge difference in any class. If you do not feel inspired and motivated in a yoga class, the teacher may be wrong with you. This does not mean that the teacher is not good in any way, but it does not help you achieve your goals.

Think about whether the teacher is teaching you the things you need to learn. No matter how good a teacher is, if he can't help you meet your needs, find another. Your best friend may be excited about her Hot Yoga class, but if it's not for you, you should look after another class. Maybe you want something less physical and more mental. There are many yoga teachers and one is the right one for you.

Are you going after your goal? A good teacher will guide you every step of the way. If you feel overwhelmed, the teacher may not be for you.

You may ask A good yoga teacher will be available to your students before and after class and will listen and respond to individual concerns. If it's not easy to reach your teacher, find one.

Feel free to ask your teacher about his training or philosophy. The best class of teachers is someone who sees yoga as a constant work of progress and is still studying with his own teacher.

This is yoga, not clothes

Do you know one of the main reasons why people don't go to the gym or stop? She feels confident among a group of perfect bodies. Yoga has become so fashionable that people are really afraid of what branded clothes are best and what color they buy.

Do you really need $ 125 Dior pants to achieve lighting? Wear everything comfortably. And don't compare yourself to others. Yoga is a personal journey. As has been said in this book, it is not a competition.

All you need for yoga is simple leggings, shorts, a tank top or a T-shirt. Seriously, you're not trying to make a fashion statement. All you have to remember is comfort. Special clothes are available for Hot Yoga. If you want the yoga mat to last, so choose a quality mat. That would be a very good investment.

Yoga classes

Other yoga classes can cost $ 20.00. It may be a supplement, but it's not scary to get you started. There are ways to practice yoga on a limited budget.

Local YMCAs, gyms and some community centers often offer yoga classes at low prices. In hot weather, yoga groups can meet in local parks. When you sign up for courses, shop in bulk. By registering for 20 lessons at once instead of individual lessons, you can get a discount.

Some yoga studios rent pads and water bottles. They can only charge a dollar or more, but additional costs may be added. Bring your own mat and water bottles from home. Some yoga studios offer "Karma Yoga" lessons. These lessons are free in exchange for studio work, such as desk management and after-lesson cleaning. If costs are a concern, feel free to ask about this option. Some studios like to sell a class for a small service.

The best time to practice yoga

It's a quick excuse not to start practicing yoga. The truth is, we're all busy. We all have the same 24-hour day. If we want to achieve something, we must devote time to it.

Traditional yoga is about sunrise or sunset. But taking the time to yoga is better than no yoga, even if practicing yoga with a full stomach is not.

good idea. Get up an hour earlier than usual and do asanas before you do anything. It strengthens and activates your body and mind in the best possible way. Physical postures can keep your body running while breathing clears the mind.

Yoga intentions

Some yoga teachers ask you to set your goals at the beginning of the program. What exactly does that mean?

It is not necessary to have an intention in order to enjoy the benefits of yoga lessons. But it can take them to the next level.

Creating your yoga intent brings yoga into your daily life. Yoga does not end when the asana ends. This should be the beginning of your spiritual journey, not its end. Yoga was originally developed as a spiritual activity. The others just follow.

The intentions explain your purpose when practicing yoga. It focuses on the personal quality you want to develop or improve. You may be hoping for more patience, knowledge or compassion for others. Maybe you want to get rid of past pain. Make it true in your mind.

Your intentions are the bridge between your poses and the rest of your life. Yoga is not like leaving the gym and forgetting about it until the next lesson. Mental exercise should be a part of your daily life. You will set your mind to be real by keeping your intentions in the spotlight. This is true spiritual growth.

Talk to your doctor before you start

It is true that anyone can practice yoga. However, before you start, you should discuss any possible restrictions with your doctor. This does not prevent you from doing yoga, but can only restrict certain movements to prevent injury. Your doctor may also have some idea of   what type of yoga is best for you. Having a doctor who has the knowledge and support of yoga is a great advantage.

Slowly and easily

If yoga is a new experience for you, then of course get excited and jump in. But the goal of yoga is not who can do the most poses in the shortest possible time. Yoga is a slow and conscious process. Each session should be dedicated to facilitating poses. Work at your own level of comfort. It is not enough to emphasize that yoga is not a competition. If some positions are harder than others, practice them until they are easier. Mastering yoga positions is not limited in time. If positions may be easier, get out of your comfort zone a bit to get to the next level, but not to the point of physical discomfort.

Start at your own starting point

Visiting a new yoga class where everyone seems to know what they are doing can be intimidating. However, this is the case when you start a new attempt.

Whoever it is, you are your own starting point. It is completely irrelevant that a person will be able to maintain the balance of one leg for 60 seconds while you continue to deviate. Areas of fear are fun to move forward as you continue. Enjoy who you are, every step of the way. Self-acceptance is the essence of enlightenment. The spiritual side of yoga promotes compassion. Start with yourself.

Chapter 09 - Preventing Injuries

Practicing yoga is as safe as walking. Injuries are therefore still possible and must be prevented.

Start by following a few basic rules. Do not practice yoga on an empty stomach and avoid alcohol. Always stay hydrated. Every yoga class should start with warm-up exercises. If you are not, find another class. As we mentioned, the right teacher can make a big difference and reduce your chances of injury. Certified teachers will go through up to 500 hours of training to obtain certification. Make sure you are dealing with a qualified teacher.

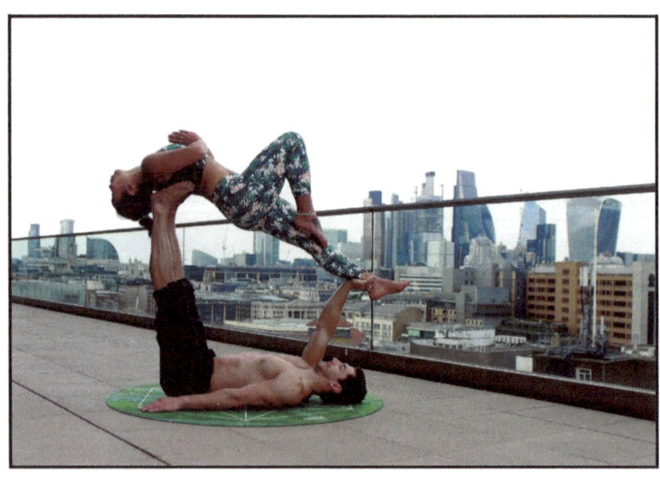

Don't try to do poses you're not ready for. This can cause severe muscle loss. Trying positions you are not prepared for is one of the main causes of yoga injuries. Know the limitations of your body and respect them. How far you go, you decide, not your teacher.

Some days you may feel more active than others. If you have a bad day, accept it and don't try the severe poses that might be possible at other times. Listen to your body. Some parts of the body, such as the neck, lower back, knees and ankles, are more prone to injury. Watch out for any poses that involve parts of the body. It is easy to get light when changing position, so always make sure you stay hydrated.

Most yoga positions can be changed with blocks or towels. Feel free to apply these adjustments until your body can facilitate the poses.

Don't start yoga by jumping into dangerous positions, such as standing on your head. This can lead to serious neck damage. Work your way to harder positions.

Chapter 10 – Yoga and Meditation

Yoga is a bridge between meditation and spirituality. Native Buddhists used yoga as a means of preparation for meditation. Meditation, like yoga itself, is mundane. Anyone can do it. The goal is to calm the loud mental conversation and calm the mind.

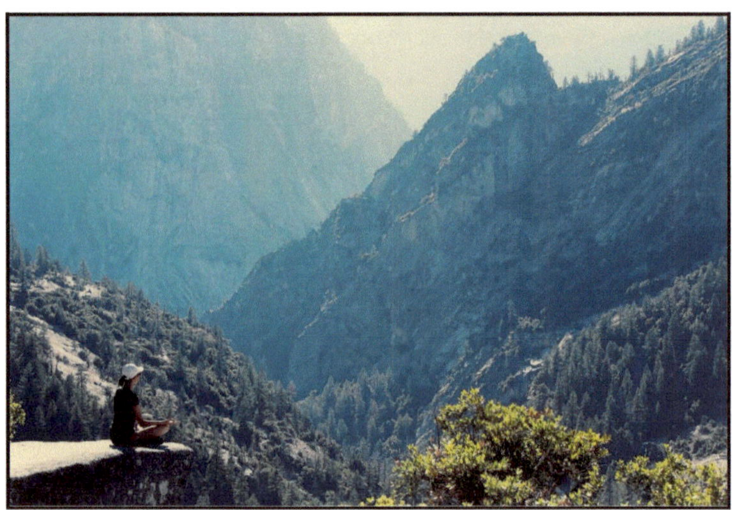

Benefits of Meditation

1. Through meditation, you become more aware of your inner and outer life. You will begin to notice emotions and thoughts that you may have denied in the past.
2. It provides insight into improving your relationships.
3. Awareness will help you move in time, instead of acting out of habit. Negative emotions can hurt you, even if you don't know the cause of your behavior. If you are aware of these feelings, you can deal with them in a positive way.

4. Meditation allows you to be less critical of yourself and others.

5. Meditation prevents you from acting on random emotions and can analyze your facts before you act.

6. Meditation can reduce stress and anxiety.

7. Meditation can help you adapt to changing circumstances.

How does meditation work?

Much research on meditation has been done in recent decades. Physically, meditation can lower our blood pressure and calm our nervous system. When we meditate, our heart rate and breath slow down.

With more knowledge, meditation can change the way we think about past experiences. If you are constantly humiliated as a child, you will begin to accept it as normal. In adulthood, you still have the same feelings deep inside you. You hope to be humbled, even though there is no reason to do so. Constant meditation can negatively change this to get you more positive thoughts and emotions.

Studies have shown that meditation can change the structure of our brain. People who meditate have improved areas dedicated to awareness and concentration. A Harvard University study has shown that while age can lower certain parts of the brain, regular meditators maintain a person's younger brain capacity for decades. For anyone looking for a higher level of existence, meditation obviously has a lot to offer.

Another Harvard study showed that with regular meditation, the areas of the brain that deal with fear and anxiety shrank, while the areas involved in empathy and compassion increased. Changing the way our brains respond means the end of control over our lives.

How to start meditation

Like yoga, meditation requires commitment. This is an ongoing process. The more we meditate, the better we will be, and there is no limit to how good we are at meditation. The ancient and modern Buddhist has spent his entire life in meditation and self-affirmation.

Meditation requires a quiet place. Most people close their eyes and focus on their breath, noticing every breath. While other ideas may be distracting, they are simply acknowledged and relegated to the sidelines in a non-judgmental way. Start with just a few minutes - it's surprisingly hard to sit still for a long time, because we're used to being active.

Work up to half an hour or forty-five minutes.

Try to meditate at the same time every day to make it a daily habit. Find a comfortable place where you will not be disturbed. Meditation after waking up in the morning can start your day positively; However, bedtime meditation can help you sleep better. Of course, there is no reason why you should not meditate for two hours a day.

Find time to meditate

Admitting that you don't have enough time is just an excuse not to start. There is no time; you can do this by getting up half an hour earlier in the morning. If you have your own office, close the door at lunch time and use time or part of it to meditate. Do you spend a lot of time on social networks? Limit your time and buy at least an hour or two every day. Thoughtful meditation

One of the most beneficial types of meditation is mindful meditation. It brings more knowledge to our minds and emotions. Many people are bound by negative thoughts, always about the events of the past years. No matter how long it takes, these emotions can still control our actions.

Mindful meditation allows us to recognize negative feelings and then reject them, so they no longer have the power to limit us. Thoughtful meditation is based on a critical axiom that cannot be too high:

You are not your thoughts.

Some people feel controlled by their negative emotions. Thoughtful meditation will give you control. Like yoga, meditation can change parts of the brain, increase our ability to relax and reduce the areas responsible for depression and anxiety.

Instead of mixing our minds with thoughts and feelings, mindfulness keeps us present to face what is happening. This is a skill that can be learned.

How to meditate intensely

Thoughtful meditation is not easy. If you can breathe, you will meditate. Follow a few simple steps and enjoy the benefits of relaxation.

Find a quiet place, preferably with natural light. Make sure you are not disturbed. If you find a quiet place outside, that's fine.

A good time for meditation is half an hour, but you can start with just five minutes and gradually increase the time. Like yoga, it should be easy and not painful or uncomfortable.

Wear comfortable clothes. You don't want anything to interfere with your meditation flow.

Helps set a timer so you don't have to stare at your watch. You can use a chair or sit on the floor with pillows. Just like on the floor, nail your feet to a comfortable lotus position, which is a traditional state of Buddhist meditation. When sitting in a chair, reach for the floor or rest your feet with blocks.

Your body should be straight but not stiff. Put your hands on your feet. You must be comfortable to relax.

Most people prefer meditation with their eyes closed because it eliminates distractions. But if you want, you can leave them open.

Then just relax. With a deep breath and exhale, slowly begin to focus on your breath. See how the air comes in and out. Feel the rise and fall of your chest.

It's only natural that your attention will wander when other thoughts come to mind. There is no reason to be angry and act like these thoughts are not. Identify them and then focus back on your breathing. If your mind wanders too much, watch what is happening in an uncritical way. Don't serve them, just pay attention to what's going on.

One way to increase attention is to count. Breathe, count 1, breathe, count 2 ... to twenty. Then count.

After completing the meditation, be quiet for a few minutes. Notice how you feel, your thoughts and emotions. Be an observer, not a critic.

Meditation is as easy as it is, but it can bring drastic changes. As you practice yoga, you will notice that your mind and body work in natural harmony.

Conclusion

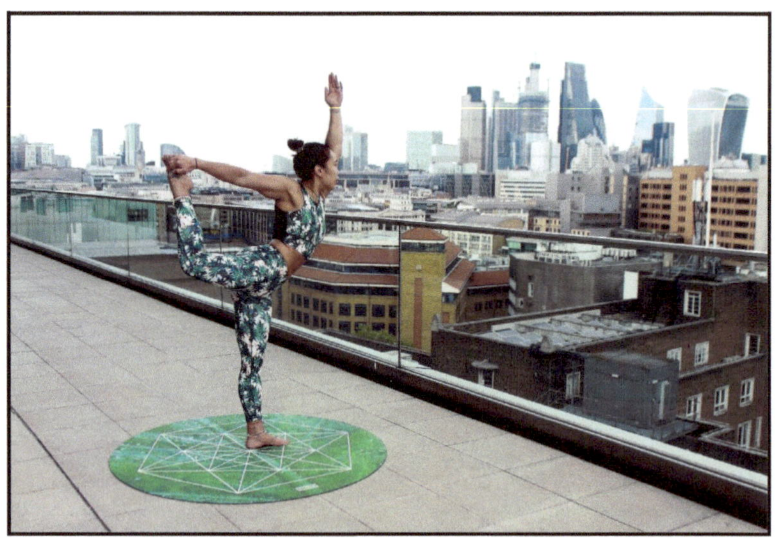

People have been practicing yoga for thousands of years and are still attracted to new practitioners, especially those in the medical profession. There is no doubt that it has something to offer when we try to reach a higher level of existence.

1. Yoga is not a religious practice. However, it brings us into contact with our spiritual mind. Original Buddhist yogis practiced yoga to increase enlightenment and improve their understanding of the world around them. Yoga is preparation for meditation. The beginnings of yoga are more spiritual than today, but they still strengthen our spiritual selves.
2. Yoga improves our immune system, heart rate, cardio, blood circulation, and respiration. Reduce stress, anxiety and improve muscle flexibility and tone. The benefits of yoga can reduce the effects of aging both physically and mentally.

3. There are many different types of yoga, some are easy and gentle, while others are extremely compelling. They all provide benefits, but we must choose the yoga that is best for us.

4. There is nothing in yoga that should be painful or forced. If you feel pain or discomfort while practicing yoga, talk to your teacher. You are doing the wrong exercises or you are in the wrong class. There are many lessons to choose from, so you don't have to deal with someone who is uncomfortable with you.

5. Yoga positions affect our entire body because it stretches our muscles to the limit. Unlike other exercises that can focus only on certain parts of the body, yoga positions involve the body as a whole. Therefore, many consider yoga to be more than aerobics or weightlifting. Aerobics and dumbbells can of course be done in combination with yoga for optical physical benefits.

6. Yoga connects the mind with the body to move the unit. We are well aware of how the mind can affect the body and our overall health. Negative thoughts can cause serious illness and inflammation, such as arthritis. The purpose of yoga is to clear the mind of negativity and restore good physical health. Remember that mind and body work together.

Use the following rules as the best way to approach your yoga sessions:

- Everyone has their own starting point, so you don't have to worry about weight, age or flexibility. Your position will improve with exercise, but it is never in competition with the rest of the class.
- ☺ Finding the right teacher can make a big difference. A good teacher should be able to answer questions and not pose poses beyond the student's abilities. If this is your experience, look for another teacher. ☺ Many people start yoga with specific expectations. But everything is different. You may not be able to take the lead while the rest of the class seems easy. That is very good. The only rule of yoga is to work at your own level of comfort. There is no need to force anything.
- ☺ Start slowly. People have been practicing yoga for decades and still strive for perfection. There is no perfect yoga position. It is only you, your body and your mind who will reach a higher level. ☺ Talk to your doctor before starting a yoga class. Yoga movements are safe and injuries are rare, but you want to make sure that nothing prevents you from practicing yoga safely.
- ☺ Meditation is an important part of yoga. As we have already mentioned, ancient yogis used yoga to prepare the body for meditation practices. To get the full physical, mental and spiritual benefits of yoga, make meditation a part of your life.

Yoga can add much to your life and can help you become a better version of yourself.

www.ingramcontent.com/pod-product-compliance
Lightning Source LLC
Chambersburg PA
CBHW040238240726
48664CB00001B/177